PUSHKIN PRESS

At the turn of the (last) century, the world was changing rapidly. Trains were faster, cheaper and more comfortable than ever before. The new craze of bicycling had given men and women unprecedented independence. And the modernisation of telegraphy and the recent invention of the telephone meant that information could be exchanged over huge distances in a mere matter of minutes.

And so a frazzled and harried world was ready for the pioneers in thinking, education and imagination to advise and instruct on the perilous "Age of Hurry". Passionate thinkers, committed campaigners, they give invaluable guidance for anyone troubled by the rush and bustle of the early century's information overload.

The books in "Found on the Shelves" have been chosen to give a fascinating insight into the treasures that can be found while browsing in The London Library. Now celebrating its 175th anniversary, with over seventeen miles of shelving and more than a million books, The London Library has become an unrivalled archive of the modes, manners and thoughts of each generation which has helped to form it.

From essays on dieting in the 1860s to instructions for gentlewomen on trout-fishing, from advice on the ill health caused by the "modern" craze of bicycling to travelogues from Norway, they are as readable and relevant today as they were more than a century ago— even if the exhortation to "never drink beer or spirits" has been widely disregarded!

LIFE
in a
BUSTLE

Advice to Youth

The London Library

Pushkin Press

Pushkin Press
71–75 Shelton Street
London WC2H 9JQ

Sir Alfred Milner, KCB, *Bustle*, delivered on January 21, 1897. (Froebel
Institute Addresses, 5). Oxford: Printed for Private Circulation by
Horace Hart, 1897

P.A. Barnett, *The Little Book of Health & Courtesy. Written for Boys
and Girls*. London: Longman, Green, & Co., 1905

Claude G. Montefiore, *On Keeping Young and Growing Old*. [The
substance of an address given to the students of the Froebel Educational
Institute, December, 1915] Reprinted from *The Journal of Education*,
March 1916

Untitled crying boy cartoon by Leonard Raven Hill (1867–1942),
published in *Punch; or, The London Charivari*, April 2, 1913

"Muddleby Junction" by John Tenniel (1820–1914), published in
Punch; or, The London Charivari, October 19, 1872

Untitled boy and old man cartoon, by an unidentified cartoonist,
published in *Punch; or, The London Charivari*, November 24, 1860

First published by Pushkin Press in 2016

9 8 7 6 5 4 3 2 1

ISBN 978 1 782272 50 2

Set in Goudy Modern by Tetragon, London

Printed by CPI Group (UK) Ltd, Croydon, CR0 4YY

www.pushkinpress.com

BUSTLE

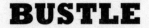

Delivered to the Students of the
Froebel Educational Institute on
January 21, 1897

BY SIR ALFRED MILNER, K.C.B.

Sir Alfred Milner's busy life as a barrister, a journalist, a private secretary to the Chancellor of the Exchequer, a Governor of the Cape of Good Hope, a High Commissioner for South Africa, a Member of the War Cabinet, a Secretary of State for War, a Fellow of New College, Oxford, a member of The London Library and a writer of history and advice on over-achievement lasted from 1854 to 1925.

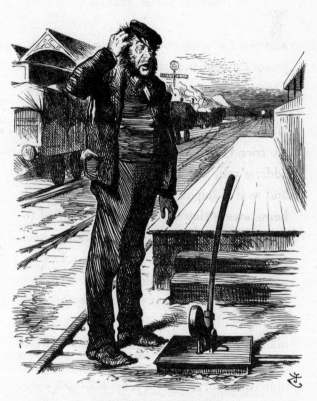

MUDDLEBY JUNCTION.

Overworked Pointsman (puzzled). "LET'S SEE!—THERE'S THE 'SCURSION' WERE DUE AT 4·45, AND IT AIN'T IN; THEN, AFORE THAT, WERE THE 'MINERAL,'—NO! THAT MUST HA' BEEN THE 'GOODS,'—OR THE 'CATTLE.' NO! THAT WERE AFTER,—CATTLE'S SHUNTING NOW. LET'S SEE!—FAST TRAIN CAME THROUGH AT—— CON-FOUND!—AND HERE COMES 'THE EXPRESS' AFORE ITS TIME, AND BLEST IF I KNOW WHICH LINE SHE'S ON!!"

I am not going to address you on the subject of Education. If that is very wrong of me, I hope you will forgive it, and, above all, that you will realize that I am not personally to blame. For my presence here to-day is due to my friend, Mr. Montefiore. He invited me to address you, and as he knows me very well, and as it is impossible to know me without being aware that I am quite unqualified to speak on any educational topic, I must assume that in asking me he intended that, whatever might be the subject of my remarks, they should not be connected with Education. And if so, I am not sure that he was not right. Nine out of ten annual addresses delivered here are likely to deal with one or other of the innumerable aspects of that great subject, which must necessarily always hold the place of honour in an institution such as this. It may be as well that now and again a casual ignoramus like myself should speak about something different, if only to serve as a foil to his predecessors and his successors. It was easy enough to see what I was not competent to talk about, but that did not take me very far. A much greater difficulty arose, when I came to ask myself about what I was competent to talk. It is perfectly clear that no man or woman has any right to stand up and lecture his or her fellow-creatures, whether in large or small numbers, on any subject on which he or she is not, in some sense, an authority. "On what subject," I said to myself, "am I an authority?" The self-examination thus set on foot was not an agreeable process. I ran over rapidly in my mind a large number of themes of common human interest in the most various fields of intellectual activity, Literature, Science, Art, Invention. It did not take me long to recognize that, despite my advanced age, I had not the faintest claim to speak with authority on any of them. This was a little daunting, but my self-respect rose to the occasion and supplied me with an excuse. "You do not pretend," it said to me, "to be a student, a man of letters, or an artist. You cannot be expected to excel in Literature, Art, or Science. Your life is one of practical business. You belong to the world of affairs." I took the hint at once, with a great feeling of relief, and began to recall to mind the numerous pies in which I have had my finger, if perchance one of these might be fit to be dished up for your information or amusement. First I tried to count up my achievements; but, alas! there was not one of them big enough to hang a sentence upon, much less a lecture. Then, in a moment of inspiration, I began to think of my mistakes. At once an illimitable field opened before me. My difficulty now became simply one of selection.

But here I was not without a clue to guide me. In questions of practical conduct no counsel is of much avail which is not based on personal experience. But the experience must not be merely individual. The errors which a man commits owing to his personal idiosyncrasy, or to circumstances peculiar to himself, are not worth his discussing with others, except possibly with very intimate friends, and then only on rare occasions. He must get over them as best he can for himself, but he had better not talk about them. To do so is mere egotism. It is almost as ill-bred to call attention to your personal defects as it is to make a parade of what you imagine to be your excellences. But the matter is different the moment the failing of which you are conscious is one which you cannot help seeing is a very general one. If the mistake you know you have made is being made all around you, it is no longer egotistical to dwell upon it, always provided you have something useful to say. If the personal experience of the most ordinary man can be made to contribute to the diagnosis of a common ailment, then it possesses an importance which the merely individual failing, even of a Napoleon, does not possess.

Now there is one mistake which I am always making, and which I can see plainly is being made by innumerable people of my acquaintance, including some of those, whether men or women, whom I most admire——yes, by women, allow me to say with all respect, every bit as much as by men. It is, I feel no doubt whatever, a failing peculiarly characteristic of our own time. The mistake I refer to is that of being in a hurry, or rather, perhaps I ought to say, of allowing oneself to be hurried. It is not so much the mere act of hurrying, as the sense of hurry, the feeling that you haven't got time, that you ought to be doing things faster, or doing more things, than, as a matter of fact, you can do. This feeling, with all its attendant evils—constant discomfort, scamped work, moral and physical wear and tear—is an endemic disease amongst us in the present age. It is not a sin. It is not a vice. But it is a very great piece of mismanagement, and we all know that mismanagement, if it is only sufficiently gross and extensive, may do much more harm than murder.

Every successive epoch of history, as we look back upon it from a distance, seems to have some dominant moral characteristic. Our own age, when our great-great-grand-children come to pass judgement upon it, will be known as the Age of Bustle. And they will note with sarcastic interest—if there is any philosophy left in those days and the excessive scurry of the previous generations has not resulted in universal shallow-headedness—that the Age of Bustle immediately succeeded, and indeed in a sense resulted from, a period of unprecedented fertility of invention, and, above all, of great time-saving inventions. Men can do now, as a rule, incomparably more things in a given time than they could a hundred years ago. They can travel to India and the Cape as quickly as their ancestors could to Rome or Vienna. They can send a message to the other end of the world in less time than it took to send one to the next county. And over and above such great discoveries as the railway and the telegraph, there are innumerable minor inventions which economize time—shorthand, lifts, pneumatic tubes, the electric light, the bicycle, the motor-car, and a hundred others. Yet the result of all this is, not that we have more time, but that we have less. You can hardly take up a paper without reading how somebody has fallen down dead with heart-disease running to catch a train, when there was another train going in ten minutes. Who ever died of heart-disease running to catch a stage-coach, though there might not be another for twenty-four hours? But then, of course, heart-disease, as well as all the nervous disorders, which are due to excitement and to rush, are almost as much on the increase nowadays as consumption and the infectious diseases, which result from want of air and insanitary conditions generally, are on the decline.

It is only another instance of the old, old story, that the actual effects of any great change of human circumstance are constantly the very opposite of what *a priori* reasoning would have led you to expect. Look at the exactly analogous case of labour-saving machinery. How many hundreds of hands does a single steam-hammer or power-loom economize? Is the army of labourers thereby diminished? On the contrary, it has been enormously increased. There is not less toil in the world, but more toil, for all the toil that machinery has taken off our hands. There is not more leisure in the world, but less leisure, for all the time which invention has made us a present of. And the reason is not far to seek. The mere fact of our being able to do more things in a given time has tempted us to undertake many more things. The time economized in one direction has been more than swallowed up by new enterprises.

Look at travel. In old days the wealthy Englishman made what was called the Grand Tour. He visited, at an immense expenditure of time owing to the slowness of locomotion, the principal countries of Western Europe. Has the fact of his being able to reach them more rapidly led to his staying longer in them and knowing them better? No. It has simply caused him to substitute the tour of the world for the tour of Europe—not to see Europe better, but to see Europe, Asia, Africa, and America—all superficially. It has produced the genus Globetrotter. Or to take another instance. In the badly paved and badly lighted streets of old London, with the lumbering coach of last century, it was as much as the lady of fashion could do to attend one rout in an evening. Now she can bowl along gaily on C-springs to three or four, but she talks dreadful twaddle at all of them. For her mind is fixed, not on what she is saying or on what is being said to her, but on nodding to fifty people in half an hour. It follows her wandering eye, while her tongue goes on mechanically without its assistance. But then, as everybody else is doing the same, it doesn't matter. Nobody listens, or could hear well if they did listen, and any individual fatuity is lost in the general babel of meaningless chatter. And then people complain that conversation is not what it was. How can it be in such conditions? The basis of good conversation is ease, repose, leisure, presence of mind, play of mind. Here you have discomfort, haste, tension, absence of mind, distraction of mind. Quantity and quality never yet could get on together, and in social intercourse they disagree more hopelessly than anywhere else.

What is constantly asserted of conversation is no less constantly asserted of

correspondence. And with equal justice.
People complain that nowadays hardly anyone
writes a good letter. That is saying too much,
but it is not too much to say that there are
fewer good letter-writers. Why? Because we
have an admirable penny post and a delivery
every two or three hours. Because we have a
cheap and ubiquitous telegraph service. What
a temptation to expand yourself in fifty different directions! So my lady dashes off ten
notes and two telegrams in the same time in
which her grandmother would have written
one letter, very carefully worded, and in the
finest copper-plate hand. This all helps to
keep up the bustle of life, but it does not tend
to promote epistolary style. Style, indeed, is
somewhat at a discount all round, especially
having regard to the tremendous amount of
our education. I admit that our ancestors were
sometimes a trifle stilted. But will not our
descendants say of us that we were more than
a trifle scrambling?

A curious and characteristic feature of
the Age of Bustle is the idolatry of mere pace,

pace for its own sake quite irrespective of any object to be gained by it. That people who are always in a hurry should be grateful for anything which takes them along quickly, is natural. But, as in so many other cases familiar to the learned, that which was at first valued as a means to an end, ultimately comes to be worshipped as an end in itself. So now we idolize pace even when there is nothing whatever gained by it. If there is one thing more than another which delights the multitude, and which spurs the ambitious youth of the day to frantic emulation, it is the "breaking of a record." And as demand begets supply in such matters, records are being broken every other week. There may, no doubt, be some value in these feats, if they are a proof of increased strength, or stamina, or agility, in the race, though as evidence of these things they are somewhat misleading. For the record-breaker is often, even physically, a very one-sided creature, who has cultivated a particular aptitude at the expense of a well-balanced bodily development and of his general health.

Still there is something to be said for doing a thing faster, if it means that your capacity of doing it has improved. But what is the use of doing a thing faster than it ever was done before, if you yourself contribute nothing to the achievement, and if the time which you save is absolutely of no use of you? There is a particular season of the year when every Londoner of properly constituted mind and adequately filled purse is in a mortal hurry to get to Perth. Not that Perth is a particularly inspiring place in itself, but it is a great distributing centre of tourists and sportsmen. Now till quite recently you could get to Perth, travelling through the night, by a train which was very fast, certainly, but not so fast as to be dangerous or uncomfortable, and which arrived at a reasonable hour in the morning. This, however, was not good enough for the Age of Bustle. So a year or two ago we invented what is known as the "Railway Race to the North." This means that you can now get to Perth by a train which goes so fast that the passengers are rattled about like dice in a box, that they are occasionally upset at Preston, and that, when not upset, they arrive at Perth, after a sleepless night, much too early for breakfast. That is progress in travelling as it is understood in the Age of Bustle.

Let me invite your attention to a similar instance of progress in another field of enterprise, which of all others is essentially modern and up to date—I mean Journalism. Ever since I can remember there has been a mortal race between evening papers, each trying to come out earlier than the other. At first they came out at three, then they came out at two, then at one; now you can get an evening paper at eleven o'clock in the morning. What is the effect of this last achievement of the great god Haste? Why simply that there is not, except once in a blue moon, any news in the evening paper which is not copied from the morning paper that you have just read— so you have merely wasted your halfpenny. Perhaps there is a tinge of acerbity in my remarks about evening papers. The truth is I have a personal grievance in this matter. I am a late riser in the morning owing to the fact that, like a true child of my age, I have been trying to do too many things overnight. When I sally forth to go to my daily labours, after a hasty breakfast, and with my nerves just slightly on edge from the sense of being late, it adds appreciably to my ill-humour—it seems an uncalled-for reflection on my habits—to have a little boy rush right into me as I step on to the pavement (of course he is always rushing to get ahead of the other little boys), and split my ears with piercing screams of: *"Star!" "Echo!" "Evening News!"* But here I feel on firm ground. I don't care what they scream. You may hurry everything and everybody that moves upon earth, but as long as old Mother Earth herself declines to be bustled, and, regardless of all the rushing and scurrying of her impatient children, still insists on taking twenty-four hours to turn round in, it never can be evening just eleven hours after midnight.

Yes, and as long as she takes 365 days to go round the sun, spring and summer, autumn

and winter will succeed one another at exactly
the old pace for all our hurrying. The corn
will take just as long to grow, the fruit just
as long to ripen. And so it is with the har-
vests of our moral life. These too cannot be
hastened. Nothing really worth having can
be got in a hurry; all thorough knowledge,
all solid achievement, almost all deep affec-
tions are the growth of years. The feverish
rush of modern life will not make any of these
quicker or easier of attainment. Indeed, if we
are not on our guard, it may make them more
difficult. Our increased command over the
forces of nature, our increased power of movement, our increased stores of knowledge—all
these advantages may be a hindrance rather
than a help, if we allow ourselves to be dis-
tracted, to be flurried, by the number of our
opportunities.

Do not let me be supposed to depreciate
the colossal progress of recent years. From
many points of view we live in a glorious
time. I have little sympathy with those who
wish they had been born at any, even the

most brilliant epoch, in the past of the human race. The Many have now opportunities of study, opportunities of travel, opportunities of healthy enjoyment, which of old were denied to all but the Few. Human activity is expanding in all directions. Life is infinitely fuller, more varied, more interesting than it ever was. But on the other hand it requires more judgement, more balance of mind, more strength of character to make the best of it. Where one can do so many things there is a real danger of trying to do too many, and the end of that is that one does nothing well. Every age has its own special difficulties and dangers. The disease which specially threatens this generation is restlessness, distraction, dissipation of intellectual and moral power. Its consequence is exhaustion and nervous collapse. And its symptom is Hurry. Where that symptom becomes very apparent it is a sure danger-signal, and its warning is: "Pull up and reorganize your life."

To many of those whom I am addressing what I now say may not come home with the force of personal experience. That is precisely why I am speaking about it. I want to tell you what is surely coming, that you may be prepared for it when it comes. I don't know if many of you are bicyclists. If you are, you will be familiar with the kindly notices which are stuck up at certain points along many of our high-roads, with the legend: "To Bicyclists this Hill is Dangerous." Well, these warnings are sometimes, I think, rather oddly located. For to be of any use they ought to be at the very top of the hill. It is not much good putting them up a little way down, where you have already begun to be run away with. And it would be of little use preaching my present sermon to people who had already been swept off their feet by the rush of active life. It is in College days, on that level plain of study and preparation, when the pace is still mainly of your own making, that it is useful, if it is ever useful, to utter the warning, that a time is coming when the pace will be made for you, and much too fast a pace unless you take care to prevent it, by external conditions. I do not say that this experience comes to everybody; certainly it does not comes to everybody in the same degree. There are useless people, whom nobody wants. They will not be dragged hither and thither by conflicting demands. There are phlegmatic people, not easily aroused to interest or moved by sympathy. These too may find time hang heavy on their hands. But I cannot believe that many of those present will have either of these two melancholy causes of exemption from the common lot of their contemporaries. And given an average amount of capacity, of interest, of sympathy—much more when all these are above the average— every year of life will increase the claims upon your time and energy. More and more will you become conscious of the force of the current which bears us all along, of the increasing strain imposed on all its denizens by the mul- titudinous activity of the modern world. And for you as for others it will become a matter of the first necessity to keep a cool head, to husband your strength, not to lose control of your own lives.

No doubt it is possible to do it. The skilful boatman can steer his course on a swift stream as surely, if not as easily, as on a sluggish one. It is all a matter of experience. Similarly, men can acquire the habit of making their way steadily amid a rushing crowd. There are thousands of people who get flustered in crossing a crowded street. But there are others who manage somehow to get across, not only with safety, but without rushing. They have learnt to keep their heads. They are not appalled by the number of vehicles. They will not let themselves be hurried, but just wait their opportunity and then pick their way as coolly and leisurely between the cabs and 'buses as if they were crossing a country lane. To the rustic who visits a great city for the first time, yet more to our occasional visitors from still uncivilized countries, to Khama or Cetewayo, the thing seems a perfect miracle. It is not a miracle, only it has got to be learnt. And many of us never do learn it thoroughly. They may not be run over, but they take a great deal more out of themselves than is at all necessary, and waste their nervous force for want of management.

Similarly, Mankind, it seems to me, have still a great deal to learn about the proper economy of strength and time in view of the increased strain of life in the most progressive communities. Fortunately "necessity is the mother of invention." The instinct of self-preservation will teach us to mould ourselves to our environment. Face to face with a new difficulty, the race will develop, as it always does, a new aptitude. Those who acquire it will prevail over the others. And in time this aptitude, which is seen to preserve life and to bring victory in the struggle, will be elevated to a place among the Moral Virtues.

May I foreshadow in conclusion what the line of development is likely to be among successful men and nations, especially in the sphere of intellectual life? The same principle will, no doubt, apply, *mutatis mutandis*, in other spheres also. But let me, by way of illustration, take study. What is the policy which the necessities of the case will force those to adopt whose aim is to attain the highest culture of their time? There is a wise old saying that we ought to try "to know something of everything, and everything of something." That puts very happily the great truth that everybody should try to be at once a finished craftsman and an intelligent citizen of the great world of thought. But what is happening every day? Why, the "something" of which you or I ought to know everything is, with the growth of knowledge, growing bigger and bigger. And the "everything" now includes hundreds of things where formerly it only included tens. But the acquisitive power of the individual man and woman has not grown—it cannot grow—in proportion. What is the inevitable consequence? Inevitably the borders of the "something" will have to be contracted. We shall more and more tend to become specialists in constantly narrowing fields. But not less on that account, nay, more on that account, shall we feel the necessity of that other form of intellectual activity, the old ideal of which was "to know something of everything." We want to see what others are doing, to bring ourselves into touch with the lives of our fellow-creatures. But the "everything" now includes so much! There is the difficulty, there is the danger. The menu is so enormous, that unless we take care we may indeed taste of many dishes, but eat little and digest nothing. Here then comes in the opportunity of our new virtue. Success will rest with those who can preserve a calm judgement, who will not be bewildered by the multitude of things offered to them, but select with tremendous rigour, and who finally, having selected, will give themselves time to enjoy what they have chosen, and not let themselves be flurried out of the enjoyment and the benefit of it by the thought of all that they have been obliged to pass by. The truth is, that we do not lose as much as we think by fixing our eyes steadily on a few points only in the vast landscape of knowledge, instead of vainly trying to take in every tree and every hedge. Those few points may be the great landmarks. Science is manifold, but the spirit of all true science is one.

He who has drawn a deep breath of that spirit from the work of one mastermind has the key to the storehouse; he has acquired the freedom of the City of Science. And something of the same kind is true with regard to the more imaginative side of literature. Books are innumerable, but the masterpieces are, after all, not so very many. And here, again, to be thoroughly steeped in the ideas of one or two of the greatest writers is in some sense to be in fellowship with them all, and with the true disciples of each of them. It is to be admitted into the great freemasonry of those who have learned to know the firstrate, and who in that knowledge have a bond of sympathy, as well as a standard whereby to measure the value of all other work. And such admission is to my mind the great object of liberal——or should we not rather call them liberating?——studies. Those who have attained it are much nearer knowing "something of everything" than if they had crammed up fifty primers, or scrambled through all the articles in all the magazines. Moreover the former process is as restful and bracing as the latter is harassing and destructive of mental fibre. For if there is one effect more than another which the highest form of work in Literature or in Art is calculated to produce, it is that of Serenity, of Repose. A great tragedy may indeed move us deeply, but it never fusses us. And it is not only the effect of the completed work which makes for calm. It is the realization, sometimes even the unconscious realization by us, as we admire that work, of all the mass of patient labour, all the controlled power that has gone to produce it, which is so steadying as well as so inspiring. Therefore I have no fear for the future of the Classics. I do not mean only the great Classics of antiquity, but the modern writers of classic stamp, our own Milton, Gibbon, Scott, Burke (typical instances these, for I am not attempting a complete list). They are so life-giving, so preservative. The men and women who cling to them will, as a rule and in the long run, prevail. And so the Classics themselves will be preserved, strengthening rather than losing their hold as the years pass. Listen, on this point, to some wise words of Matthew Arnold. "Even if good literature," he says, "entirely lost currency with the world, it would still be abundantly worth while to enjoy it by oneself. But it never will lose currency with the world, in spite of momentary appearances; it never will lose supremacy. Currency and supremacy are ensured to it, not indeed by the world's deliberate and conscious choice, but by something far deeper, by the instinct of self-preservation in humanity."

Selection, therefore, the rigorous and patent adherence to the few best, the refusal to be torn hither and thither by the many little, is certainly one side of that yet nameless virtue which Mankind has got to develop, and which is going to preserve the Elect in a world of Bustle. But there is another side to that virtue, less lofty perhaps, but not less necessary——a knack, if you will, rather than a moral grace, but still of immense importance if we are to escape Hurry and all the nervous wear and tear which it involves. I mean the knack, so rare, yet so invaluable, of providing yourself with a Reserve of Time. Economy of time, in the sense of always having some time to spare, some time in hand, is essential to the successful conduct of life in a society like that in which we live, so busy, so hurrying, so full of unexpected calls upon its members. The importance of a Reserve of Money is apparent to everybody. Who is well off in respect of money? Does it depend only upon the number of hundreds or thousands a year? No, whether a person is really well off depends far less upon the amount of his total income, than upon that of his margin for unforeseen requirements. You are not rich with £10,000 a year if every penny of it is required for some inevitable item of expenditure. You are not poor with £100 if you have £10 to play with for odds and ends. What is the essence of good finance? In framing a Budget, whether for an individual, a household, or a State, the great, the vital point is to leave that ample margin for the unforeseen. You may estimate your expenses ever so carefully, yet, unless you provide for the chapter of accidents, you are sure to come to grief. If your contemplated expenditure does not leave something over for the unforeseen, then cut down that expenditure. It is bad, it is fatal finance to have nothing in hand, for the only thing that can be safely asserted of the unforeseen is that it is sure to happen. And precisely the same rule should apply to your Time Budget, as to your Money Budget. In making your plans of life, in laying out your time, always leave a margin, an ample margin, for the work which is not in your programme, for the calls upon your interest, sympathy, assistance, which you cannot foresee. If the work you have undertaken is bound to take up the whole of your time, you have undertaken too much. Reduce the number of your engagements. And that for two reasons which apply to Time just as much as to Money. Everything, as a rule, costs more, in Time as well as in Money, than even upon a reasonable calculation it is expected to cost. We are all too sanguine in that respect. And then, in addition to the excess of expenditure on the known, there is the great chapter of the unknown. Unless these two things are borne in mind, what will happen? Why, you will not only be absolutely on your beam-ends if some sudden emergency arises, but you will be always behindhand, always in a hurry, even with your ordinary business. I know people, scores of them, who are very proud of themselves when they have filled up every hour of their day. Their idea of saving time is to cram the maximum number of jobs into a given number of hours. There is one piece of business at ten o'clock. Half an hour is estimated for that, so something else is put down for 10.30. That is, perhaps, a little more formidable, therefore it is given three-quarters of an hour. Next job, therefore, at 11.15, and so on through the whole list of available hours. What happens? The very first thing proves a little more difficult than was expected. It turns out that it cannot be properly done in only half an hour. Therefore one of two courses must be adopted. Either you must give it three-quarters of an hour, and thereby disturb your whole carefully arranged programme and be late at every moment of the day, or else you scamp it, do it in a hurry, do it badly. Of all the detestable men to do business with is the man who has made up his mind beforehand just how long to give you, and who, whatever new, unexpected and important points may turn up in the discussion, cannot extend that fixed allowance. Finally, something happens requiring your attention which was not provided for at all. That breaks down the whole scheme, and chaotic flurry reigns supreme.

On the other hand, with a margin you can never be wrong. It is ten to one you will want it. If not, what could be more glorious than to find yourself in possession of more time than you had counted on? Of all luxuries I know few equal to the unexpected collapse of a business engagement through no fault of one's own. A present of time! Why, it is like an unexpected legacy. For what man or woman who really lives, and does not simply vegetate, in this world of ours—this world so full of interest, of movement, of novelty—has not a hundred things that he wants to do, things to read, to see, to hear, if only Time were not wanting? Just think of all the things you want to do some day or other. How pleasant to find yourself unexpectedly free to do any one of them! Except in moments, happily rare in most lives, of great unhappiness—a misery that gnaws at the heart and for which work may be the only palliative—how great a privilege it is to have a balance to your credit in the book of Time!

Yes, for the healthily constituted mind there is always something to be done with Time, as there is always something to be done with Money. If you don't want it yourself some one else is sure to want it. What a benefactor of society is the man capable of work, yet endowed with leisure. How many posts there are unfilled, how many duties unprovided for! And let us not neglect the claims of a healthy and recuperative idleness. Time can seldom be ill spent, if you are that way inclined, in lying on the grass, provided it is dry enough—a large assumption, I admit, in a climate like ours. It can seldom be ill spent, again if you are that way inclined, in sitting with your toes on the fender and building castles in Spain. If you really enjoy either occupation, it is a pretty sure sign that it is good for you, much better than fussing about and making work, which is not really necessary, as a sacrifice on the altar of Bustle. In my experience it is just the people who enjoy lying fallow, who are capable of the most intense and effective energy when any real call comes.

The great thing, after all, is to know when to summon all your forces into the field, to mobilize your reserves, if you are wise enough to have them, to bring to bear your whole unexhausted strength upon some work of vital importance. The demon of restlessness is always at our backs, tempting us to fritter our strength away. "See how short life is," he whispers. "The time is ebbing. Bestir yourself, work, bustle, or you will be left behind in the race." Yes, work by all means, steadily, patiently, adding to your knowledge, harvesting experience, building up your strength for the day of trial. But don't make work. Don't bustle. There is lots of time if you don't waste any. You cannot hasten Opportunity. Sooner or later it comes to most of us. The great point is to have your resources well in hand to seize it when it comes. No doubt there are people who, in common parlance, never have a chance. That is Bad Luck. But there is one thing worse than never having a chance, and that is to have a chance and to have squandered beforehand the power of using it. That is Failure. You cannot provide against Bad Luck. But you can provide against Failure. And there is no commoner cause of Failure than Impatience. "Work and wait."

THE LITTLE
BOOK OF
HEALTH AND
COURTESY

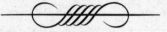

Written for Boys and Girls

BY P.A. BARNETT, 1905

PERCY ARTHUR BARNETT (1858–1942) grew up in the Jews' Hospital and Orphan Asylum, Norwood. As well as being a member of The London Library, he was a teacher and educational theorist, and was sent to oversee the reorganization of the education system in Natal following the Boer War. His daughter, Charis Ursula Frankenburg, became a pioneering writer on birth control, and his son was killed at the Somme.

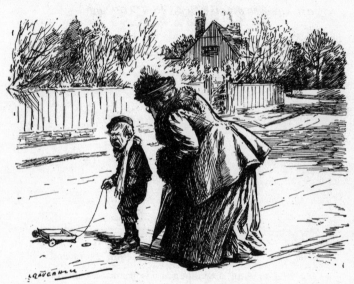

"I SHOULDN'T CRY IF I WERE YOU, LITTLE MAN."   "MUST DO SUMFING; I BEAN'T OLD ENOUGH TO SWEAR."

"No decent person uses bad language."

The kingdom of heaven is... of those who are easy to please, who love, and who give pleasure.

R.L. STEVENSON

It is sometimes thought, and sometimes even said, that a person's manners matter very little if only his character is good. This is a mistake. It is true that a man may be a good man and yet be rough in manner; but his goodness will "go further," it will be more useful both to himself and to others, if he makes himself pleasant to other people.

The reasons why we are expected to do some things and to avoid others are not always clear to us at first sight; but we should think twice and thrice before assuming that no reasons exist. Customs are often the result of the wisdom of many men and women, and have come into use because somehow they have been found to make the business of life easier and pleasanter; or because they serve to protect us from thoughtlessly slipping into actions or habits which are harmful.

* * *

THE REAL ROOT OF ALL GOOD MANNERS IS GOOD FEELING. TEACH YOURSELF TO BE KIND.

* * *

Our first duty to others is to be healthy and cheerful. We must keep ourselves as clean in person and in clothes as our work allows us to be; and if our work soils us, we should carefully clean ourselves and our clothing when it is over. Dirty boys and girls do not rest as thoroughly as clean boys and girls; and they are very unpleasant companions.

* * *

Night and day the windows should be open. To breathe the same air again and again, as you *must* do if the used-up air is not carried away and fresh air brought to you, is unclean. Our bodies throw off waste matter, and if we breathe this into us again instead of getting good fresh stuff to take its place, the whole body becomes weaker and very soon diseased.

The bad effects may not show themselves at once, but they are perfectly certain to come.

* * *

Bed-clothing should be warm but light; feet should be kept warm. The pillow should not be too high; if it is, you cannot breathe properly.

* * *

When you rise in the morning, the bed-clothes should be thrown right back, so that the air may get to them. The bed should not be made immediately, or it will be wanting in freshness and comfort.

* * *

Before leaving the bedroom, see that nothing is left lying about which can be put away into its proper place by yourself. If servants are to come afterwards to "tidy up," it is kind and proper to save them trouble. If no one is to come, and you have to see to your room your-self, you will the more easily find things again if you put them always in the same place.

* * *

Once a day the whole body should be washed. If you cannot get a bath, sponge yourself and then rub yourself down with a towel. For the daily wash it is best to use tepid or cold water; but once a week the body should be soaped and washed in warm water.

* * *

Every morning, before washing your face, try to open your eyes for a moment or two in tepid water.

* * *

Carefully clean the ears inside and at the back.

* * *

Brush your hair well *with a brush that is not too hard*. The use of a hard brush, though it freshens you up, often tears out the tender hair and will make you bald before your time. After combing your hair with a comb that is not sharp and pointed, clean the loose hairs from your hair-brush, and then clean the comb itself with your nail-brush. Few things are so disgusting as a dirty comb.

* * *

If you have been using a washing-basin or a bath which is to be used by others also, leave it perfectly clean and ready for the next person. Let the water run out, and see that no traces of your use are left to offend him. Put soap and brushes away. Take with you to your own room your towel, sponge, tooth-brush, tooth-powder, and all things reserved for your own use.

* * *

There are certain duties connected with the cleanliness of our houses, our clothing, and our bodies, and with the removal of waste, which are sometimes performed for us by other persons; but there is nothing done for us by others which it would degrade us to do for ourselves. To think that we should be degrading ourselves by performing unpleasant duties, and to think at the same time that others are degraded by performing them for us, is mean and base in a double degree.

*   *   *

Learn how to do as many things as possible for yourself.

*   *   *

Teeth should be cleaned morning and night; *but especially at night*. Many people lose their teeth quite early in life because they do not remove small particles of food which ferment between their teeth during sleep. It is particularly necessary to clean the teeth at night after drinking milk. Whenever possible, the mouth should be thoroughly rinsed after a meal. With many people, otherwise quite healthy, food ferments very rapidly if left in the mouth; and they become unpleasant to their neighbours without knowing it. In using a tooth-brush remember that the back of the teeth must be cleaned as well as the front. Do not use a toothpick in the presence of other people.

* * *

From an hour to half an hour before breakfast drink at least half a pint of water. This helps to clean the inside of the body, and supplies it with some of the moisture which it needs so much. Doctors tell us that most people drink far too little clean pure water.

* * *

After washing your hands, see that your nails are clean. But neither pare your nails nor use a pocket-comb except in private or in places where you can offend no one else.

* * *

If others are not rising as early as yourself, make as little noise as possible; and if you are down first, look round to see whether there is any little thing that you can do to save trouble,—even if it is only to cut bread and set chairs.

* * *

Go to bed as early as you can.

* * *

Never drink beer or spirits.

Table Manners

It is a great offence against good manners to come to table unwashed and unbrushed. Eat slowly and take small mouthfuls. To see a person "wolf" his food is not pleasant. It reminds one of a wild-beast-show at feeding time; and, besides, victuals that are swallowed without being well chewed clog and crowd the body and end by doing more harm than good.

* * *

Do not speak when your mouth is full of food.

* * *

Eat soup and drink liquids quietly.

* * *

Keep your lips closed on your food. The "click-click" of food in the open mouth is a very disagreeable sound. It is not necessary that the mouthful should be seen when it has once passed your teeth; the lips are flexible enough to allow the work of the mouth to be done without much show.

* * *

It is even more disgusting to hear people suck their teeth after a meal. If the teeth need clearing, leave the company of other people and use a tooth-pick.

* * *

Do not begin your meal with a long drink. If you must needs drink at meal-time, wait until the middle, or, better still, the end of the meal.

* * *

Do not lift up your fork to plaster potatoes or other things upon it. Keep it low, and raise it only when it has received all the load that you intend to lay upon it, which should be a very moderate one.

* * *

On no account should the knife ever be raised to the mouth. Even cheese, which was once allowed to travel on the knife, should be pressed by the knife on to a piece of bread or biscuit and so conveyed to the proper quarter.

* * *

Before drinking, place knife and fork on your plate; and lay them side by side when you have finished.

* * *

Do not take large helpings of salt or mustard or other such things, nor make an ugly-looking mixture of the different things on your plate.

* * *

When you are helping yourself to food, do not take too large a share.

* * *

If there is no one present whose special duty it is to remove plates that have been used, get up quietly yourself from your chair and remove the plates of an older person or a guest, without fuss or clatter.

*   *   *

See that older people and guests are well supplied with all that they need, but do it quietly. In handing things about the table, be careful not to be so hasty as to knock the taller articles down, and be especially careful in pouring out liquids.

*   *   *

Do not place elbows or arms on the table. Sit up without stiffness or slouching.

*   *   *

Pull your chair close enough to the table, and your plate and cup near enough to yourself, to carry food to your lips without risk of spilling it.

*   *   *

Do not leave the table without asking leave, or until the rising of some older person whose example you may follow.

* * *

If you want any particular thing that is not within your reach, see where it is, and ask the person nearest to it if he will please pass it to you. Do not cry "Sugar, please!" to the wide world, and expect every one to look round for what you are pleased to want.

* * *

A saucer is meant merely to steady the cup and to catch stray drops; you may not drink from it.

* * *

Do not fidget with the things on the table. If you are not using them for practical pur-poses, "Hands in the dark" is a good rule to remember.

* * *

The tea spoon may be used to stir the tea or coffee in your cup; but when this is once done, lay the spoon in the saucer, and do not be con-tinually stirring with it or drinking from it.

* * *

Older people, who do not always sleep well at night and often have worries which boys and girls cannot understand, sometimes prefer to have as little talk as possible at breakfast. Be cheerful and happy in the morning, but not boisterous or noisy at table.

* * *

Talk at meals should be about pleasant subjects.

In the Street and Travelling

Everybody is entitled to use the street; but only in such a way as will not interfere with the comfort and business of other people.

* * *

Look where you are going. If you want to stop and gaze at something, get quietly out of the way of those who do not share your desire.

* * *

Carry your stick or umbrella point downwards.

* * *

On a narrow or disagreeable path a man who is walking with a woman takes the less pleasant side. He leaves the pavement to let a woman pass, whoever she may be; and if he is walking with a girl, or woman, or some one much older than himself, he walks on the outside, nearest the kerb-stone.

* * *

If several friends are walking together, they must be careful not to take up all the path. Ample room should be left for others to pass, in whatever direction they may be going.

* * *

No kind person allows orange-peel or banana-skins or other slippery matter to remain on the pavement; and only a selfish blackguard throws a lighted match where people are walking or passing.

* * *

In a crowded or narrow thoroughfare keep generally to the right. In towns, where so many people pass through the streets, we cannot say "Good morning" or "Good evening" to every one that we meet; but in country places such a kindly greeting is very pleasant both to the giver and receiver. It makes both more cheerful, and makes the world feel friendly.

* * *

Remember that public places belong to everybody, and that no one has the right to make them unpleasant for others. Do not therefore eat strong-smelling things in railway carriages, nor litter such places with waste-paper, fragments of food, fruit-skins, and the like. Find some spot where you can stow such things out of sight without offence.

* * *

Do not shout or "rag" in railway carriages, nor talk loudly in any public place about affairs which interest only yourself and your friends.

* * *

On entering or leaving a railway carriage always quietly close the door after you. This will earn you the silent thanks both of the passengers and of the busy guard and porters.

* * *

None but "cads" deface or destroy public property. No decent person cuts or writes his name, or anything else, on things which are not his own; nor does he put his dirty boots on public seats.

* * *

Do not crush your way into a carriage; boys and men should see that women and girls and old folk come to no harm.

* * *

Spitting in public streets and carriages is not only filthy, but also dangerous to public health.

* * *

Avoid hideous snorts and sniffs in clearing the

air passages of nose and throat. If a handkerchief is useless for your purpose, go for relief to some private place where you will be a nuisance to nobody.

* * *

If you cannot help coughing or yawning, turn your face aside and cover your mouth.

* * *

Never giggle or talk in such a way as to make people think that they are the subjects of your mirth or conversation.

* * *

If strangers or elderly persons come into a room where a boy chances to be wearing his hat or cap, he should at once take it off; and if a boy anywhere meets some one to whom respect is due, he should not be afraid to show the same mark of respect. Take your hat right off; do not merely lift it sheepishly.

* * *

Learn to shake hands heartily. Your hand should neither grip like a vice nor should it lie in the hand of your friend like a deceased fish.

Books and Writing

Use books, and especially other people's books, carefully. When you handle a book, see that your hands are clean. Finger-marks in a book are sure signs of slovenly and even dirty personal habits.

* * *

Turn over by carefully lifting the page *at a corner*, and never wet your finger for the purpose. If pages stick together, blow them apart.

* * *

Do not put your fingers to your mouth when you are reading or thinking, and never bite your nails.

* * *

If you wish to keep your place in a book, do not turn down the corner of a page, nor lay the book flat on its face. A strip of clean paper will do all that is needed, and will not disfigure the leaf.

* * *

Sign your name clearly. It is a foolish kind of vanity to make a signature which people cannot easily read. In the same way be careful that the address from which you write and the address on the outside of your envelope can be read without trouble. Think of the postman.

General

Close doors after you, but close them gently. Do not let them slam.

* * *

Rub your boots or shoes on the doormat before entering the house, and then, if you are at home, change into dry clean shoes. It is a good plan to change stockings or socks at the same time as boots.

*   *   *

If by any chance you get into another person's way or otherwise cause him unintended inconvenience, say "I beg your pardon," at once, and do anything that is possible to set the matter right.

*   *   *

If some one, in like manner, has cause to make this slight apology to you, the proper form of reply is "Not at all." This does not mean that the apology was not necessary, but that the offence is no longer remembered.

*   *   *

If somebody has made a mistake against which you had warned him beforehand, do not say "I told you so." This is ungenerous, and useless as well; for it irritates your friend, and, unless he himself is very sensible, may prevent him from profiting by the lesson which his mistake brings with it.

* * *

Girls are sometimes given to make foolish little parties and little secrets amongst themselves for the mere purpose of keeping other girls out. This is silly, and may cause much pain.

* * *

To be rude or unkind to people over whom you have any sort of power or authority is very base and hateful. You must be equally courteous to every one. The use of "Please" and "Thank you" is not really mere empty form; it means that you do not desire to give trouble, and that you are grateful for services rendered to you, however small.

* * *

To make fun of people unkindly or to jeer at them is a mark of meanness. And if another person has done something which both you and he know to be wrong, do not "nag"; that is, do not continually remind him of it. If he is young enough and you are old enough, a few kind words will do much more good.

* * *

Make the best of everybody. To find fault is one of the easiest things in the world. Grown-up people whose duty it is to look after others have to check and guide them, and sometimes to rebuke them. But every one, and boys and girls especially, should make the most of the *goodness* of people, and should be ready to believe that people mean well rather than ill. As a matter of fact, they *do*.

* * *

Speak up, and look at the person to whom you are speaking; and do not, in conversation, continually address him by name.

* * *

To be shy means often that you are thinking too much about yourself. Do not make yourself uncomfortable by thinking that others are criticizing you.

* * *

Show no desire to pry into places or things which do not belong to you, or to know about the affairs of other people when they do not directly concern you. And even when they do or may concern you, wait until you are duly informed. You must not force yourself into a conversation nor ask that the subject of it should be explained to you. Wait till you are addressed.

* * *

Carefully avoid even glancing at letters or other papers belonging to some one else. If letters are given to you to post, you have no right to read the addresses.

* * *

Do not talk of disgusting subjects even with people whom you know very well. If such subjects are often in your mind and on your tongue, you will at last become so familiar with them that they will not offend you, and you will become coarse without perhaps knowing it.

* * *

No decent person uses bad language. It is easy to hold yourself back from such things, even when you are angry; and in controlling your tongue you gain command over yourself in other ways. You will avoid not only *saying* what you may afterwards be sorry for, but you will also avoid *doing* it.

* * *

When bad words or talk are used in your presence, quietly go away. Do nothing to encourage them. If you cannot get away, remain silent. If those who offend are of your own age, you should say plainly that you do not like such things. If the offender is a boy or girl younger than yourself, it is your duty to rebuke.

* * *

Do not tell unkind tales about other people, whether your telling causes punishment or not. If your talk is about other people, tell things about them that will make them better friends of those with whom you are talking. Tell people of the *kind* things that are said about them; and if nothing kind has been said, tell nothing. It is a wicked thing to kill others' happiness, and this is what the mischief-maker does.

* * *

Be on the look-out to offer any little service you can to women and elderly people—indeed to any whose sex or weakness or age gives them a claim upon you. Open the room door for them if they are leaving; help them with coat or jacket; put them comfortably on their way; see them safely to tram or train. But do it all without fuss—to serve *them*, not to draw notice on yourself.

* * *

Never interrupt a person who is speaking. Listen quietly till he is finished, and listen as if you were interested. If you wish to add something, or to correct a mistake into which he has fallen, do it courteously, and not as if you were anxious to show how much better informed you are than he.

* * *

Never bandy words with an angry or unreasonable person. Remain silent, or answer gently. Do not quarrel.

* * *

"Calling names" is useless, foolish, and rude. Only vulgar people "call names."

* * *

Englishmen pride themselves on "playing the game," that is, on being fair to every one. Take a beating in your games just as you would behave after a victory—quietly. If a point is disputed, hear everything that the other side has to say; and if there is no umpire or referee, consider it carefully. But always uphold an umpire, and play a losing game as cheerfully and as hard as if you were winning.

* * *

Be very slow to take offence. "Touchy" people are mostly vain people. Even though folk may seem unkind, it is better to think that they do not mean to annoy you. Remember that you yourself may have hurt the feelings of some one else at another time without meaning any harm; so give them the benefit of the doubt. If they do in fact mean to wound you and yet do not make you angry, they will soon tire.

* * *

Whatever happens, do not whine. A grumbling discontented person is of no use to anybody. He is, indeed, a general nuisance, for he makes every one uncomfortable. Put a good face on things, and draw profit from misfortunes by taking them as lessons.

Be cheerful and *look* cheerful.

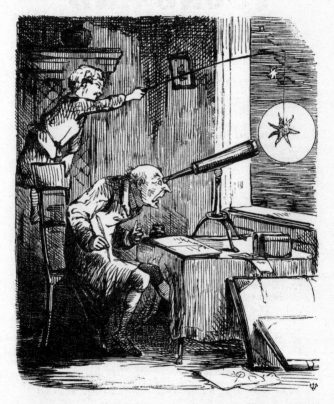

"Admiration keeps up young. It is connected, on the one hand, with pleasure; it is connected, on the other hand, with wonder."

ON KEEPING YOUNG AND GROWING OLD

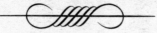

*Delivered to the Students of the Froebel
Educational Institute, December, 1915*

BY C.G. MONTEFIORE

The scholar, philanthropist and reformer CLAUDE
JOSEPH GOLDSMID MONTEFIORE was a member
of the Anglo-Jewish elite who broke with Jewish
orthodoxy when he founded Liberal Judaism in
Britain. He died "disappointed and embittered" at
the relative failure of Liberal Judaism, which he
blamed on the rise of Zionism. After his death in
1938 The London Library received a bequest of all
the pamphlets (around 5,000 titles) he had collected
in the course of his life.

I propose to talk to you this afternoon in a quite informal way, as a friend who may claim the privilege of intimacy in a college which he has known from its foundation. The "young" and "old" of my title are obviously to be understood in a figurative sense. Literally, all of us, if we live, must grow old. Yet, as I hope to show you, there are ways whereby we may both keep young in heart and mind, and grow old in another sense than merely in days. Old age, as the author of the Wisdom of Solomon reminds us, is not merely "that which stands in length of time," nor is its measure merely reckoned "by number of years."

Most of those I see before me are, in the most literal sense, still young. Youth is with them to make or to mar. But I do not propose to speak directly about the right way in which to spend it. There would, indeed, be much to say about work and play; the joys and sorrows of youth; its responsibilities and its limitations. For though many of us look back to our youth as the happiest period of our lives, yet in the perfect, or ideal, life we may rightly hold that each period of it, even old age itself, has its own special satisfactions and achievements, perhaps even its own peculiar joys. And, if youth is rightly used, there is the greater chance of a happy maturity and old age.

> *Grow old along with me!*
> *The best is yet to be,*
> *The last of life, for which the first was made.*

So what I want to speak about is rather the future than the present, less of youth itself than the passing of it into manhood and womanhood.

In a peculiar sense, you who are students in this place are standing at the parting of the ways. When you leave us, we, who are grey-headed and fairly aged, shall think of you as still very young. But if, in a year or two, you are in the thick of teaching, or if perchance

74

you are married, with a house of your own, you may say, "It seems an age since I was at college"; or even, "I begin to feel ever so old." And, indeed, in a certain sense, the period of youth will be over, the period of womanhood will have begun.

The seven terms of this college life are a sort of prelude, a busy pause, a delightful in-between. Such at least was the college life which I knew myself long ago: one was no longer a boy: one called oneself a man: and yet the strain of real manhood had not quite begun.

To each period of life, as I have said, its own glory. Alas! it is not always so, as we know very well, and one of the objects of this very college is that there may be a larger proportion of glorious childhoods—so far as wise education and admirable educators can secure them. And even to a right and happy childhood, and a right and happy youth, there may not always succeed a right and happy womanhood, or a right and happy old age. Life may be cut off prematurely, or circumstances may prove too hard, or a peculiar individuality may fail to find its proper nurture and environment. But while we admit, and seek to make ourselves prepared for, the shocks and uncertainties of life, there are yet castles in the air which it is right and wise to build ourselves and to encourage others to build likewise. We can, to some extent, make the ideal real—real to us and part of our inner selves. Even what we would *have*, we can sometimes help to procure; still more what we would *be*, we can, to some extent, make ourselves. We have a margin of power; we are, within limits, "captains of our fate." Shall we, then, ask what would we fain be in character, and what powers of heart and mind we would possess, when we are, or if we become, forty or fifty or sixty years old—a long way off, as it must seem, to most of those present here to-day?

The answer to this question is implied by my title. All of us would fain achieve the wisdom of age, and also retain the heart of youth. And one may add at once that, as experience shows, this wish is not impossible of realization. For there are, indeed, radiant souls, both men and women, who possess this desired combination: the wisdom of age and the heart of youth. We may even vary and intensify the phrase, for we may say: the wisdom of age and the heart of a child.

Let us consider a little more closely what we mean by "the heart of youth," "the heart of a child." We are thinking to some extent of the actual child, but more of the child as poetry and romance and even religion have pictured him.

There are many ingredients in our meaning. Some are very deep and solemn things, and some are light and airy things, yet all make the same or very similar demands on those who would acquire them. There is the saying which, to almost all of those here present, comes with the accents of authority, that the very passport or key to the Kingdom of Heaven is to become as a child. Something deep and solemn must here be meant, and the reference is less to any actual child than to the ideal child. And in our list of meanings we should also come down to such apparently simple things as the capacity to enjoy like the child, the capacity to laugh like the child.

"The wisdom of age and the heart of youth." The combination implies a demand. To obtain it means a demand upon us in each direction of our nature, and certainly in three—a physical, an intellectual, and a moral demand. Just a word as to the physical demand, by which I mean the discipline of the body and the care of health. Let me read to you some sentences of a great teacher upon this subject:—

Among the responsibilities of youth which I hardly know whether to call greater or lesser, for it is very great if we consider the consequences and the punishment, but not so great if we think only of the moral fault of neglecting it, is the care of health. It is a duty of which we hardly think, and had better not talk: it is one at which we may sometimes be disposed to laugh. For in youth most of us have health enough and to spare, and we cannot look forward thirty or forty years to a time when the remains of it may have to be husbanded. We do not keep before our minds life as a whole, in which there are many things to be done requiring our whole strength, or remember that there is one condition of success in any business or profession, and that is good health. And in almost every case it is in our own power to secure this.[*]

I would add to these weighty words the reflection that, though we have all known persons who have triumphed over the weaknesses of the body, and who, in spite of constant ill health, are young in heart and mind, yet ill health—bad digestion, nerves, or whatever it may be—makes it more difficult to remain young or grow wisely old. We are strange combinations of body and mind and soul. And no

---

[*] Jowett, *College Sermons*, page 141

one can afford to say: "I can neglect my body without detriment to my character or to my mental and moral powers." Overwork and carelessness about food and rest may lead to many evils, both mental and moral: and among these evils may be that, even metaphorically, youth may fly away, and the wisdom of age may not appear. "Work hard, but don't overwork," is the counsel I would offer you, and this, as I shall try to show, is no empty paradox.

I am thinking not so much of your college career as of the many years which I hope are to come after college life is over. For those years I would say, "Be careful not to let the mind rust." Do not be content with the modicum which will get you through your teaching or your household duties. Add, if you can, by effort just a little more. I would not advise people to read what is clearly too difficult for them. One must recognize one's own limitations. We get no profit from a book which is unquestionably beyond us. To be able to make a quotation from Spinoza or Kant or Plato looks learned, but may be a purple patch or worse.

But I would advise that, if possible, during the year one should read or re-read (perhaps often only re-read) a book which is quite up to the level of one's own capacities or just a very little bit beyond them. You may remember that in his delightful *Talks to Teachers*, William James lays down the rule: "Keep the faculty of effort alive in you by a little gratuitous exercise every day." On the purely intellectual side, I would not go so far as to say, "every day," but I would, at all events, say: "sometimes," or "occasionally"! It will help to keep you young. And for those who are going to become teachers, I would combine James's maxim with some advice of the great Teacher (in the more general sense of the word) whom I have already quoted.

One good method of keeping young is not to regard one's education—even one's education from books—as finished with one's college career. One may wisely continue, as this high authority recommends, to study from the speculative side the profession in which one is practically engaged. Or, again, we may keep a little time in the vacations either for a subject which, though distinct from, yet connects with, our daily employment, or for one which, perhaps, furnishes the greatest contrast to it.* In one or other of these ways we may seek to keep our minds fresh and strong and keen.

But now let me allude to something deeper and more fundamental—something which affects both our intellectual and our moral life. She, then, who would wish to keep young, and grow wisely old, must retain, and, if possible, increase, her power and her capacity to admire. For admiration keeps us young. It is connected, on the one hand, with pleasure; it is connected, on the other hand, with wonder. And being connected with wonder, it is also connected with the supreme quality of reverence. If you admire, you will almost always feel pleasure in that which you admire. To be able to feel keen pleasure in right and noble things and persons is a mark of wisdom and of

---

* Jowett, *Dialogues of Plato*, Vol. III, page ccxi (Third Edition)

youth—of that youth which may be combined with age. It keeps us young to continue to feel pleasure in croquet or chocolate, but far more to be able to admire. Take, for instance, the love for, the pleasure in, and the admiration of, scenery or pictures or music or poetry. Not all of you can, or can deeply, or can honestly, care for all four of these. Let us suppose you honestly care for two of them. It is of great importance to keep up the power of caring for them by exercising it. If you keep the capacity, you may even increase the degree, and you may, in all probability, be able to increase your judgment and discrimination. It is, therefore, worth while to take a little trouble to seek, or not to neglect, opportunities for maintaining and exercising our power to admire.

Let me here say a word, by way of example, about the care for poetry. I would urge those who can honestly say that they admire and find pleasure in poetry to find time to read some good poetry every month or two months. It need not necessarily be fresh poetry; it may often fitly be the poetry which they have already read. Let them also, if they can, maintain the power of learning a little poetry by heart. If we do not care for poetry when we are twenty, we shall hardly care for it when we are fifty or sixty. And note this. The great poetry which we are able genuinely to care for at twenty, we may, with exercise, continue to care for at fifty. But not all of us may be able at fifty to learn to care for any great poetry which we did not already care for at twenty. Our minds often become less flexible as we grow older: most of us become, in some ways, more conservative. Learn, therefore, to admire some of the immortals when you are young, and if you do not neglect them too utterly, you will retain the capacity to admire them—you will even admire them more deeply, more intelligently—when you are old.

No less important than the retained capacity to admire things is the capacity to admire persons. Youth is said to be the season for hero-worship, but if we want to keep young, that worship must persist all through our lives. And not merely hero-worship of the immortals or of public men and women still living, but also hero-worship for some persons whom we ourselves know. The word "hero-worship" may, however, be misleading to some of you. It may suggest something affected, sentimental, or foolish. I do not mean anything of that kind. I mean rather the power to appreciate, to realize, and to admire human greatness and human worth, or even a sweet and gracious, a pure and noble, human personality. I mean the power to feel before the human mind and before human goodness a certain reverence, a certain awe. Youth is, or should be, the age of hero-worship, but it is too often the age of criticism, and, at worst, of cynicism. I would venture to warn you against the dangers of such a temperament. One danger is that it make you unwisely old. I admit that we may pour forth admiration towards a particular person, and that he or she may turn out unworthy. The shock of discovery may do us harm. But, nevertheless, the risk is worth running. We are very unfortunate if we have not met four or five persons—they may be within our own families, or both within and without them—whose boots we should not think it an honour and a privilege to black. It is quite true that we may sometimes mistake a goose for a swan, and I have admitted that, if we discover our error, the shock may do us harm. But far worse than the error of mistaking a goose for a swan is the error of mistaking a swan for a goose. That error shows just that lack of capacity within ourselves which prevents us from keeping young and from growing wisely old.

Admiration depends upon two primary qualities: reverence and humility. The conceited person and the person who, whether in man or nature, finds nothing whereat to marvel and show reverence, will soon grow unwisely old. The world has nothing to offer him; how can he keep his heart fresh and keen if that heart has nothing to admire, to reverence, to love? He cannot fill his heart except with self: so filled, it is really empty. And the empty heart grows quickly old. Admiration, on the other hand, keeps the heart employed. It is "a shield and a buckler" against the days of evil and adversity. It maintains buoyancy. It is not only a consolation, but also a stimulus. Admiration makes us believe, in spite of disappointment and sorrow and failure, that beauty and wisdom are realities, that they are among the things which are best worth living for. But above all, admiration makes us believe that righteousness and goodness are realities, both on earth and beyond earth. They, above all else, make life worth living: they, above all else, make us strong and keen in the conviction that it is worth while ourselves, so far as in us lies, to do and to be good. Cheap cynicism and cheap conceit—these are the two vices which, above all other vices, prevent us from keeping wisely young and from growing wisely old.

Connected with the capacity of admiration, but yet distinct from it, is the capacity to feel and to be genuinely interested in ideas, movements, persons. So far as persons are concerned, this capacity to feel interested is allied to the quality which we know as sympathy, about which I have no time to speak. But I must say a few words as to the maintenance of interest in movements and ideas. Here, too, for most of us, a certain effort will be needed. First, we shall need it in relation to our own study or business or occupation. What seemed true and good in 1915 may receive several hard knocks in 1930. Or, though still true and good in its measure, it may need supplementing, or even superseding, by something truer and better. Nevertheless, we may prefer to keep to the old routine and the old ideas. To suspect that what we had regarded, and yet regard, as gospel truth is very doubtful, and that the methods we had deemed, and deem, so valuable and adequate are, perhaps, unwise and insufficient, is very painful and disagreeable. Many of us prefer to shut out newer light and to draw down blinds over the windows of our minds. But these blinds will make us dull and sluggish; they will tend to turn us into fossils. There are fossils at thirty, and there can be living and growing organisms at sixty. So let us keep our powers of interest well awake and often used.

Yet to you, to whom this particular fault has not yet come, I must add a warning. There are two opposite evils, both of which we must seek to avoid. It is not well or wise to be moved away from old moorings too rapidly. It is not desirable to be blown about by every new wind of doctrine; immediately to catch on to, and bow down before every new fad and eccentricity, or even every new theory and method. Formed convictions with a willingness to learn—that is the ideal, but it is not an easy ideal, whether in education or in theology. St. Paul said, "Prove all things; hold fast that which is good." But this advice or maxim is not within the power of us all. We cannot prove, or taste, or inquire into, or study, all things. We have not the time. One must be willing to make a selection even in one's own subject. And, on the whole, it is wiser to know a few masters and masterpieces in education thoroughly than to attempt a feeble knowledge of many. And one has to remember that a theory or a method may be new—perhaps even it may be the rage—and yet it may be only partially true. One does not keep rightly young by becoming a person who hops rapidly from one fad to another. On the other hand, one must not be afraid of the new, and, above all, not afraid of it because it is irksome or unpleasant. One must keep the power alive to appreciate, or even, if necessity arises, to study, the startling, the novel, the upsetting. And this power one must try to use and keep alive even in regard to subjects which lie outside one's own particular occupation or profession. For nobody should have no interests except in her own mission or calling; else she is likely to become narrow, obtuse, and wooden. Least of all should a teacher have no other interests than her own craft, not merely because a teacher must be the very last person to be narrow, obtuse, and wooden, but also because education touches so many other subjects. Politics, ethics, history, psychology, philosophy, sociology, and religion——all have their bearing upon education. It is abundantly clear that no one can seriously study, or even read books about, all these vast subjects: few can seriously study, though it would be well for every teacher to have a modest or bowing acquaintance with, some one of them. Yet it is no less clear that we must all form some opinions about political, ethical, and theological matters: our minds cannot, and should not, be a blank, neither can we keep them in complete suspense, concerning these great subjects. What, then, is to be done? More especially what is to be done so that here, too, so far as our limited powers and opportunities go, we may keep rightly young and grow wisely old? I would suggest that we, at all events, maintain alert the feeling and the conviction that great problems and mighty questions are involved or contained in these subjects, full of interest and complexity. We need by no means suppose that in politics, morals, and religion, everybody is equally right and equally wrong, but I would ask you to combine your own definite and even firmly held opinions with an interested and tolerant mind. New ideas, discordant judgments, may not by any means be necessarily true; nor, on the other hand, because they are agitating or troublesome or uncomfortable, need they be necessarily false.

The young in years are by no means always tolerant of the ideas of their elders when these ideas seem narrow and old-fashioned; but the old who are also young may learn a tolerance, or, rather, a certain sympathetic understanding and appreciation, of the ideas of yesterday, and the ideas of to-day, perhaps also of the dawning ideas of to-morrow. And of one subject—the greatest subject of all—I would observe that the wisely old who is also wisely young—she who has the true heart of the child as well as the wisdom of age—will agree with the saying of a great Englishman that it is "a source of calm and repose" (shall we also add, of youth and strength?) "in our religious life always to turn from small things to great, from things far away to things near at hand, from the foolishness of controversy to the truths which are simple and eternal, from man to God."*

---

* Quoted by Jowett in his great sermon on Baxter as from Baxter's autobiography. I have not been able to find it there. But even if it is Jowett's own, the words "great Englishman" equally apply (*Biographical Sermons*, page 80).

Shall we now seek to sum up what we have so far said? How to keep young is one of the ways in which to grow rightly old. We desire to retain the youthful heart and the eager, youthful mind, but also to acquire that large, developed, and wise heart (for there is a wisdom of the heart as well as a wisdom of the head), that stored and sensitive and tolerant mind, which is characteristic of a good old age. Therefore, in the words of the Psalmist (according to the excellent rendering of the Revised Version), we still may pray: "So teach us to number our days that we may get us an heart of wisdom." Perhaps it may be usefully added that this heart of wisdom—this not purely intellectual wisdom—is to be partly obtained by active doing as well as by thinking and study. Some practical work, if the stress of teaching or of household cares allow time for it, will be of great advantage to us through all our lives, apart from the help we may thus render to others.

Our instruments, our organs must be rightly used in youth that they become not rusty in age. Keen of heart and mind; not ignorant of evil, but with a still greater conviction of good: such would, and such should, we be.

Once more we ask: How is this ideal to be realized? And once more, one is bound to reply that to a large extent no words of another can help us. Each must shape her own life: each, alas, must make her own mistakes, each must fashion her own experience. Each of those here present, if she lives and looks back upon her life after forty or fifty years have passed away, will wish that in several things she had acted otherwise; neglected opportunities, wasted or ill spent hours, will crowd upon the memory. Yet to know beforehand that this universal experience will also be ours need not, and should not, discourage us. Though all are bound to fail somewhat, a measure of success is also possible. Thus an attitude of combined seriousness and cheerfulness befits us, as we look forward into the hidden life that lies in front, and awaits us. A good deal is in our power, and of our moral, and to some extent, of our mental, future——if I may so express myself—we have, in some measure, the control. If those whom I see before me to-day live till they are sixty, few among them—I hope it is not rude to say this—will be very wise or even exceedingly good. Yet with moderate fortune, it may be within their own power to keep themselves, or to become, alert rather than dull, sympathetic and interested rather than wooden and obtuse, humble and receptive rather than conceited and self-satisfied, helpful and joyous rather than gloomy and apathetic. In the art of keeping young and growing wisely old, the cleverest among you had better not be over confident, but the least clever need have no reason to despair.

PUSHKIN PRESS—THE LONDON LIBRARY

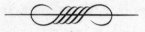

"FOUND ON THE SHELVES"

1 Cycling: The Craze of the Hour
2 The Lure of the North
3 On Corpulence: Feeding the Body and Feeding the Mind
4 Life in a Bustle: Advice to Youth
5 The Gentlewoman's Book of Sports
6 On Reading, Writing and Living with Books

FORTHCOMING:

7 Through a Glass Lightly: Confession of a Reluctant
   Water Drinker
8 The Right to Fly
9 The Noble English Art of Self-Defence
10 Hints on Etiquette: A Shield Against the Vulgar
11 A Woman's Walks
12 A Full Account of the Dreadful Explosion of Wallsend
    Colliery by which 101 Human Beings Perished!

THE LONDON LIBRARY (a registered charity) is one of the UK's leading literary institutions and a favourite haunt of authors, researchers and keen readers.

Membership is open to all.

Join at www.londonlibrary.co.uk.

www.pushkinpress.com